SLEEP...
when I want
... where I want

Olivier Pavie

Table of contents

PREFACE

One of our difficulties of our life is always to be always on the move, whether for your home or business, friends or association activities … If we add to this some everyone's health problems, life may appear tiring.

I personally travelled a lot, as many people as you will say. I also worked a lot with shifted hours, for periods of up to several weeks. I am not unique either. But I have to say that I am a man of solutions.

At that time, I had a very active family life. My three children were very young. I also needed to be an active involved father as I was working 14 hours a day, awaken at 3 am and going to bed from 9 pm to 10 pm. I had three main activities: I earned a living writing books in the IT field and new technologies, I was a journalist in this same field and I provided multimedia consultancy services.

Writing is not so easy, in computer science a little bit less. Maintaining a peak mental ability during so much time had forced me to think about improving my sleep, to get a better sleep.

It has taken me a few years to improve my technique. Even if finally, it is quite simple… Once to get used to. It is like biking, once you have learnt, you use it when you want, even if you did not practice for years.

What made me decide to write this method / book is because of all the people I have seen around suffering from a lack of sleep. People who are told about the vertues of the microsleep without any explanations about how to experience it with efficiency.

Stewardess and stewards' comments have also convinced me: they never had seen somebody like me sleeping such a long time. I had the compliment after a flight between San Francisco and New-York: asleep before the take off and awaken after the landing. Another time between Paris and the island of Saint-Martin in the Caribbean, I woke up with a blanket put over me, looking at the passengers who were disembarking. I don't even remember when we took off and I did not put the blanket over me! Living in the south of France, I often go from Nice to Paris and inversely, it takes me only a few minutes to sleep when I want it… In short, it works out well almost all the time. And if I say almost, it is mostly because sometimes I forget about using my technique. On the other hand, sometimes, I choose to think instead of sleeping. Some other moments I choose to keep my imagination wandering until I decide to sleep. Awaking, I remember that I choosed to stop wandering in order to sleep with my technique. From time to time, it takes me two or three attempts before I sleep: Too many thoughts in my mind

This book, very simple, very short, will try to explain to you the technique that I developed that can be enriched by the peculiarities of each. I will describe several examples of situations in which I use this technique so that you can better understand the "concept" or "philosophy". From this approach, either it will work directly on you, or you will imagine and develop variants that improve the efficiency of the technique for you. For sleep, there are not only ready-made truths.

A TECHNIQUE COMING FROM A SONG

The first lyrics of French singer Claude Nougaro's song "Le Cinéma", "On the black screen of my sleepless nights," inspired me one evening. Black / white, sleepless nights, dream ... In my head, it's been a trick : "on the white screen of my black nights". That is what you have to see! White as a white light ! The idea seemed bright. It is, in a way, but it's still more subtle than that. And there is work in project mode!

This project mode is what I will focus on. Because you will see white light, but not at all in the form of a beautiful all-white screen.

Second clue, the white light we talk about a lot for people coming back from deep coma or "death" : the intense white light at the end of a tunnel. We are getting closer to the concept. The moment I really advanced faster in improving my technique was when I managed to isolate a fundamental element of the basic techniques of self-hypnosis that my grandfather Robert had explained to me when I was a teenager ; relax your body, get rid of all the tensions that you feel when you go from bottom to top focusing mentally.

I also can say that I amplified the effectiveness by adding a breathing technique that was combined with all the other techniques I had started to assemble.

Finally, what is also important is to make welcoming the place where you want to fall asleep. It can be a mental posture like feeling we love the place. It may be to think of putting a cushion or a pillow to better hold the head ...

All this end to end looks like the cabin of a car: a steering wheel, pedals and a shifter; it's all about driving well by coordinating all of this.

REMOVE TENSIONS AND CONCENTRATE

In absolute terms, finding the right time to fall asleep does not exist, even when one is exhausted! It takes the mind that goes well to go out like that. This is the problem that affects everyone that the title of this book has called, and of course many others who think that falling asleep is just natural and must happen when it should happen.

Learning to take care of oneself and thus to adjust one's "sleep" time becomes an imperative when clocks can no longer stall sleep periods with the reality of life.

So let's start with some exercises to "feel" the sensations that I want to get you to coordinate in order to reach faster the real restorative sleep.

I use this term of exercise to better break down the bricks of the method I developed. It is the combination of these bricks or pieces of the sleeping machine that defines the method.

EXERCISE 1: CLOSE EYES AND RELAX

Situation:

The easiest place to start doing this exercise is simply your own warm, cozy bed. When you master the whole technique, be aware, that even the seat of an airplane or a car passenger seat, without turning it into night mode by lowering the backrest, is just as effective as a good bed.

I am not talking about train seats, which are usually either with totally fixed backrests or with folders that lower themselves by pulling the seat towards the front.

In both cases, choose the position that best suits you as shown below.

Difficulties: to concentrate

Allotted time: about 10 minutes for each different sitting or sleeping situation. For this first exercise, try three situations until you feel what is required.

Exercise:

The idea in itself is quite simple:

1. Put yourself in a comfortable position

   - Rest your head in a position that will not bother you if you fall asleep.

     .

     - o If you are used to snoring and waking up, put yourself in a position on the side instead.
     - o If you are on an airplane or train or car seat, lean your head to one side so that your falling asleep does not cause a fall in front of the head.
     - o If you have support on one side of your seat, use it in the way you feel most comfortable; possibly by creasing a scarf, a sweater, a blanket between the head and the support (window, porthole ...).

- Place the rest of your body in a position that will not bother you too. I mean that there are positions that can cut off the circulation of hands, arms and it must be avoided. Your body must be relaxed, without constraints other than the limits of the place you occupy. In a bed, it's easier than on a seat. In this last case:

  - Arms on the armrests can block circulation on the elbows and wrists.
  - It is best to put your forearms on your thighs, your thighs slightly apart, your hands falling almost between your knees.

2. Close your eyes, relax and check that your body does not seem to have a tight position.

- With your eyes closed, quickly review the relaxation of your feet, legs, arms, hands, shoulders and head.

- You seem comfortable, try to relax the tensions of your face as much as possible. Try to loosen all the tension in your eyes, including around, to minimize the pressure of closing your eyelids.
  - To check that your eyelids are closed, ask your eyes to go slowly from right to left then from left to right as if they were open, while remaining closed eyelids.
  - Do not do it ten times, two to three times are enough to feel the maintenance of the eyelids that does not require special effort, but just their natural rest.

Important: repeat this exercise several times in different sitting or sleeping situations. The goal is to feel this relaxation in a body well installed by controlling the relaxation of tension around the eyes.

EXERCISE 2: OPEN EYES UNDER EYELIDS

Situation:

For this exercise, you can be wherever you can sit for a few minutes while being able to close your eyes. If the place is public and you are shy, consider closing your eyes is a natural gesture that allows to rest the eyes a few seconds or minutes and that is really good. Try to find a relatively peaceful place to concentrate a minimum.

Difficulties: find a place where you feel good to close your eyes from a few seconds to a few minutes.

Exercise:

Generally, when we close our eyes, we do not become aware of the position of the eyes under the eyelids. Except sometimes on the beach where we will perhaps close the eyelids and slightly open them to see the sun's rays or the blue sky without sunglasses and without hurting the eyes.

1. First, close the eyelids.

2. Try to hold your head upright as if you are looking far ahead.

3. Try to find out if your eyes are actually looking away: to do this, open and close your eyelids quickly. You should see instantly in front of you. Your eyes are well oriented to watch while your eyelids are closed.

4. Practice several times until you feel well when your eyes are wide open behind the eyelids: this position of the eyes behind the closed eyelids is that which maintains a minimum tension. The eyelids are just laid.

Important: this exercise is mandatory, it serves to improve its concentration and will serve thereafter.

EXERCISE 3: COORDINATION OF EXERCISES 1 AND 2

Situation:

I do not give the details of the whole situation. As we use a method that requires concentration, I tell you where you are: you have reached point 2 of the situation of the exercise 1. Put yourself in the situation that you most appreciated during this exercise.

Difficulties: master exercises 1 and 2.

Exercise:

- Your eyelids are closed, you are in a totally relaxed situation (exercise 1).

- Do as in Exercise 2, act as if you are looking ahead keeping your eyelids closed.

- Make sure you do not have tension around your eyes, this can cause shivers related to a perception of great physical relaxation. If you have the sensation that these shivers want to manifest, let them act, the sensation is a well-being.

- Try to watch what your eyes see. Obviously, with the eyelids closed, nothing concrete but games of shadows and lights in shades ranging from black to copper (red) through gray variations. Perhaps you can see clearer shades related to the bright atmosphere of where you are. Perhaps you can see what your imagination is projecting on your eyelids.

EXERCISE 4: LOOKING FOR WHITE/LIGHT

Situation: for this exercise, you must prepare as in Exercise 1. You can also be in the case of exercise 3, but not necessarily. Here, concentration is important: let the mind open to situations of white, whitish "lights" that appear in your eyes. White is a goal, not an end in itself.

Difficulties: it requires a good concentration.

Exercise :

If it's not always easy to concentrate on understanding what to do in this exercise, a good way is to be in the dark for a few minutes then to display the smartphone screen for 2 or 3 seconds then turn it off. The persistent light in your eyes is frankly white or paler, and takes only part of your sight. It is therefore superimposed on the black and materializes clearly. Close your eyelids without tension, keep focusing on this light.

In this exercise, the goal is to be able to focus the longest on this trace in order to continue to see this white at all costs.

Obviously, this white tends to be transformed; the white rectangle left by the screen of the smartphone decreases its size until becoming a circle, a comma, a ghost ... Concentrate on following this transformation, follow the variations in brightness of the white.

It's a pursuit / hide-and-seek game. If you test this situation several times, you will start manipulating this white brightness. It will mix with unknown images that will appear. They will be supposed to represent situations, landscapes, characters, objects ...

You will have the impression of consulting an encyclopedia of the imagination. Stay focused on the white, the ideal is to reach an intense white light, a bit like the end of the tunnel whose light you can see from the outside, dazzling. Look at it !

If you can not see enough of this white, continue to follow the images that are drawn and continue to explore for white, for light.

EXERCISE 5: LEARN TO BREATH BY RELAXING EYES

Situation: when we sleep, we usually have a regular breathing whose sound serves as a lullaby. Put yourself in the comfort situation of exercise 1. And if you know that you snore in certain positions, put yourself in a position that does not make you snore or almost. In general, the position on one side or on the stomach stops snoring. All this comfortably...

Difficulties: the easiest exercise.

Exercise:

- Once in the comfort situation, with the eyes simply closed, start to breathe slowly in a rhythmic way 3 to 4 seconds of inspiration, 3 to 4 seconds of expiration.

- To stay well relaxed, choose the breathing mode that causes you the most physical ease: breathe through the nose, breathe through the mouth, or even inhale through one and exhale through the other.

- The concentration must be on the rhythm which must be very regular; for that, listen to your breath while you control that your eyes have no tension.

- You feel like a fullness invading you.

EXERCISE 6: SLEEP WHEN I WANT WHERE I WANT...

We come to the implementation of the final method that combines all the exercises described above. We will call this method Exercise 6, to continue to keep clear references. This exercise can be practiced only for the purpose of really wanting to fall asleep, with all the conditions to make it work as previously described in this book.

There are four main situations:

1. Sleep normally in bed ;

2. Sleeping in a displacement situation already mentioned in previous chapters ;

3. Sleep for a real restorative nap ;

4. Sleeping in the case of a micro-nap.

For the last two cases, some tips to optimize the time and gain a real rest.

Nap

The nap is a special moment. One decides one's will, for one's pleasure, for one's rest at a time of the day when one is in good mood: usually after lunch, when the digestion begins, which undoubtedly tires.

Napping is the happiness of Weekends, holidays, retirement for some. The nap is at home, in bed, in the couch, in the lounge chair or the hammock in the garden, at the beach. We breathe the happiness of knowing that we go to bed and that we will wake up when the body decides it, or if something external decides to put an end to it: the cries of the children, the spouse who decides that it is time to wake up, a fig that falls on you because under the fig tree was the best place ...

A good sleep for the nap will always be restorative. It is best to take advantage of it.

The moment being well chosen, the situation must be too.

Mini-naps and micro-naps

Micro-naps are very restorative in terms of sleep. And above all, they are made to enjoy a moment of fatigue that must be optimized at best because it is short. The technique defined and explained in the previous chapter is typically the right solution for this optimization. There are, however, some basic precautions to be taken to ensure success.

Make sure you are in a place of true calm without the risk of being disturbed during the time allotted.

Sleep when I want

Situation:

The question is: where to start? It's simple, everything starts with the relaxation situation of Exercise 1. What is very important is that exercises 1 and 4 are under control; the search for white must have already been fruitful. You can also start from this situation and add the other exercises as you go along.

Difficulties: depends on efforts made during previous exercises.

Exercise:

- Put yourself in a comfortable position;

- Close your eyes, relax by checking that your body does not seem to have a tight position;

- Try to release all the tension in your eyes, including around, to minimize the pressure of closing your eyelids;

- Open your eyes wide behind closed eyelids while controlling the tension around your eyes;

- Look straight ahead then sweep in search of white or light;

- Start your rhythmic breathing by continuing to control the tension around your eyes and looking for white and light: the slightest spot a little lighter projected by your imagination on the eyelids can be your driver;

- Use your eyes and mind to play with the space you create and enter to find white, light;

In this situation you are in the conditions to fall asleep. If you feel that your mind is coming out of this situation of looking for white and light, start concentrating again by checking globally the situation in which you are:

- o *Ensconced;*

- o *Without tensions in the body and around the eyes;*

- o *Concentrated on looking for white, closed eyelids and eyes wide open behind;*

- o *Concentrate on your breathing rhythm as you listen.*

Sleep... when I want... where I want

THANKS

My warm thanks to Michelle Auzolat who played the game to test my method and asked me to continue this book project and its future developments.

Sleep... when I want... where I want

www.ingramcontent.com/pod-product-compliance
Lightning Source LLC
Chambersburg PA
CBHW051407280526
45784CB00007B/3132